# Eliminate Pain!
## How to get rid of arthritis and joint pain Naturally!

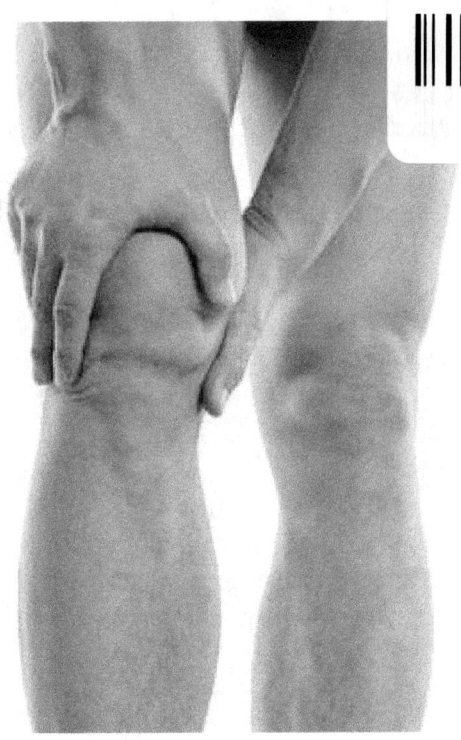

I0420321

**By M. Usman**
**Health Learning Series**
**Mendon Cottage Books**

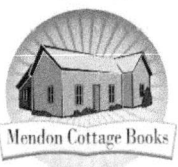

*JD-Biz Publishing*

## Download Free Books!
## http://MendonCottageBooks.com

**Disclaimer**

The information is this book is provided for informational purposes only. It is not intended to be used and medical advice or a substitute for proper medical treatment by a qualified health care provider. The information is believed to be accurate as presented based on research by the author.

The contents have not been evaluated by the U.S. Food and Drug Administration or any other Government or Health Organization and the contents in this book are not to be used to treat cure or prevent disease.

The author or publisher are not responsible for the use or safety of any diet, procedure or treatment mentioned in this book. The author or publisher is not responsible for errors or omissions that may exist.

**Warning**

The Book is for informational purposes only and before taking on any diet, treatment or medical procedure it is recommended to consult with your primary care provider.

### Our books are available at

1. Amazon.com
2. Barnes and Noble
3. Itunes
4. Kobo
5. Smashwords
6. Google Play Books

# Table of Contents

# Introduction

Are you worried about your arthritis problem? Is arthritis pain ruining your life? Does it make you feel useless and handicapped? Do you wish to live a healthy and normal life again? Now arthritis is not an issue of mystery anymore because it can be cured and treated well.

All your questions, concerns and queries are going to be answered through this book "How to get rid of arthritis and joint pain naturally." This book will give you a brief review of all the possible causes and treatments of arthritis. The book will provide you guideline regarding the lifestyle changes, eating habits, medical treatment, surgical treatment and natural remedies for arthritis. Having a detail look of this book will help you overcome the arthritis within no time.

# What is Arthritis?

Arthritis is an inflammatory disorder of joints in which the joints become painful, taut and stiff. Incidences of arthritis and other joint disorders have been increasing for the past few decades. Almost every other person suffers from joint pain at least once in his lifetime. Growing number of arthritis patients has drawn the attention of people and medical sciences towards this important issue.

Several questions might pop up into your mind regarding arthritis like, "What is arthritis? How do the joints get inflamed? What are the possible causes of arthritis? For having a proper understanding of arthritis, one must know about the normal structure or anatomy of a joint. A joint is point or place in body where two bones meet. Joint are responsible for whole body movements, so when bones rub against each other during movement there are high chances that friction might develop between them. But nature has provided a protective mechanism in the form of cartilages. Cartilages are layers of tough, elastic and fibrous connective tissue which cover the surfaces of bones making a joint. Cartilages prevent the rubbing of bony surfaces against each other. Another protective mechanism to reduce friction is the production of synovial fluid. Joint capsules are lined by "synovial membrane or synovium" which secretes synovial fluid in joint cavity. Synovial fluid is a slippery fluid which acts as a shock absorber during movements.

Whatever the reason or cause of inflammation is it results in tearing of cartilages and decreased production of synovial fluid. So, when the bones in an inflamed joint rub against each other, a high friction is offered. This makes the movement of joints difficult and the patient complaints of pain, redness and tautness.

# Types of Arthritis

More than 100 types of arthritis have been identified. Let us review some important types of arthritis which are seen commonly.

## Osteoarthritis:

Osteoarthritis is the most common type of arthritis. The basic cause behind this type of arthritis is the wearing and tearing of cartilages covering bones. It is also known as "degenerative disorder of joints". Rupturing of cartilages increases the friction between bones, leading to pain and swelling. Osteoarthritis most commonly occurs in weight bearing joints such as knee and hip joint.

## Rheumatoid arthritis:

Rheumatoid arthritis is a systemic, autoimmune disorder in which antibodies are formed against the body tissues. Normally, the defence mechanism of body provides protection against invaders by forming antibodies against them. But in autoimmune diseases the healthy and normal body tissues in body are  recognized by defence system as foreign bodies and the antibodies are formed in response which attack and damage the normal tissues. Rheumatoid arthritis affects soft tissues and joints. Degeneration of cartilages and bones leads to swelling and pain. Rheumatoid arthritis commonly affects the joints of hands, feet, elbow, neck and shoulder.

## Gout:

Gout is condition characterized by deposition of uric acid crystals in joints. In gout there is a disorder or a defect in metabolism of uric acid, resulting in deposition of needle shaped crystals of uric acid in joints. Uric acid accumulation evokes an inflammatory response which is manifested by damage of joints and pain. The commonly affected joints by gout are big toe, knee joint and wrist joint.

Gout

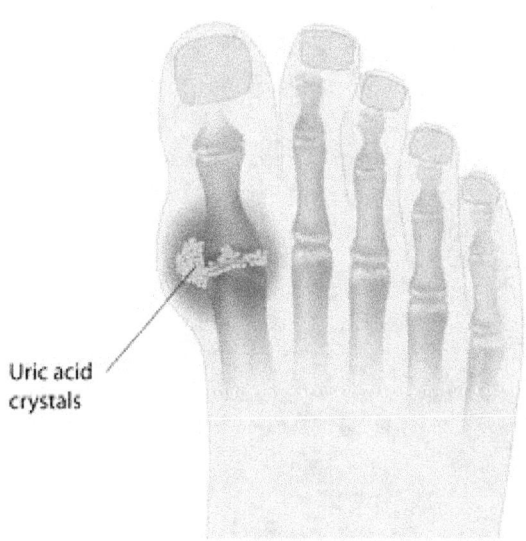

Uric acid crystals

### Infectious arthritis:

This type of arthritis arises due to bacterial infection. Bacterial infection causes inflammation of joint and damage of bones and cartilages, leading to pain.

## Psoriatic arthritis:

Psoriatic arthritis is an inflammatory disorder of skin characterized by formation of scaly, itchy, dry and reddish patches on skin. Psoriasis not only affects skin but also affects one or more joints, causing their inflammation. It is observed that patients suffering from psoriasis often complaint of joint pain. Psoriatic arthritis affects joints of toes, fingers and spine.

# Symptoms of Arthritis

These are the most common symptoms associated with arthritis.

- Pain.

- Tenderness.

- Warmth .

- Stiffness.

- Swelling.

- Redness.

- In osteoarthritis the joints are usually stiff during morning time.

- Pain in joints while walking or doing any work is an important sign of osteoarthritis.

- Loss of flexibility.

- Reduced motion of joints.

- In rheumatoid arthritis the joints are involved bilaterally and symmetrically. For example if the elbow joint of one side is affected the elbow joint of other side will also be affected, sooner or later.

- Pain, swelling, stiffness and fatigue are more pronounced in case of rheumatoid arthritis with the involvement of fever and rashes.

- Inflammation or swelling of fingers and bid toe is the typical sign of gout related arthritis. Joints are painful, taut, warm and red.

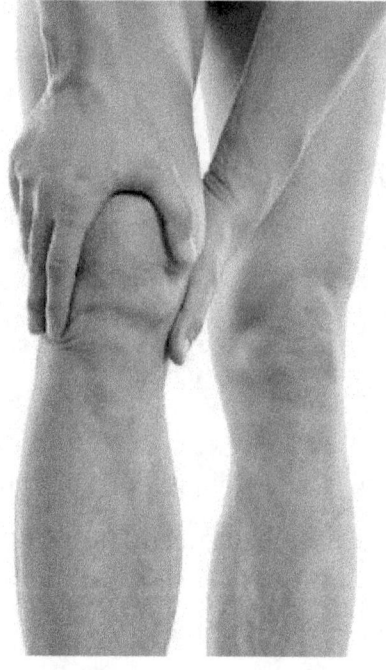

# Causes of Arthritis

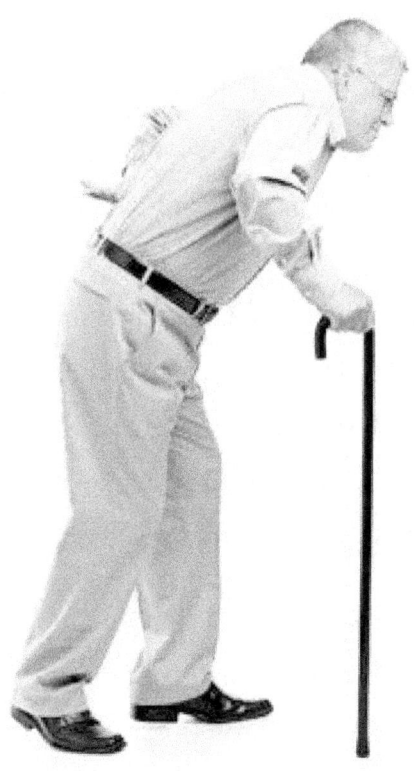

**Age:**

Aging is a natural and inevitable process. Aging is the bitter fact of life and its consequences are undesirable. Arthritis or joint pain has a deep connection with age. Aging is process in which degenerative and regressive changes start in the whole body. Joints and bones are mainly targeted in aging. As the age progresses, cartilages become brittle and bones become weak, soft and porous. Wearing and tearing of cartilages and decreased production of synovial fluid makes it difficult for joints to move, leading to pain and aches.

## Sex or gender difference:

Sex and gender difference also affects the incidence of arthritis in people. Women are more susceptible to arthritis and joint disorders because their bone density and strength is less than males. In women pregnancy also affects the bone strength. So, multiple pregnancies and mineral deficiency in mothers may lead to weakening of their bones. Postmenopausal women are the targeted victims of arthritis because the levels of estrogen hormone, needed for maintaining bone strength, are too low in them.

## Hereditary:

People who have a family history of arthritis are at the high risk of developing joint disorder and pain. Genetics always play a critical role in appearance of any disease. Same is the case with arthritis because if you have strong family history of a disease, you are more likely to have that disease in your lifetime.

## Obesity:

Research has shown that obesity has profound link with joint pain. Sometimes joints are damaged when extra load is put on them. Weight gain puts pressure on weight bearing joints of body, making them prone to weakening, damage and arthritis.

## Injury:

Injury or trauma to bones and joints increases the risk of arthritis. Chances of injuries are high in sports person such as baseball pitchers and tennis players. Heavy sports put strain on joint and may lead to their dislocation and inflammation.

## Infections:

Arthritis can be the outcome of any bacterial, viral infections or the deposition of substances like uric acid crystals. Infection causes inflammation of joints and in turn, activates the immune system of body. Persistent infection or illness over activates the immune system and as a result the healthy tissues and joints of bodies are also affected by antigen induced antibodies.

# Home Remedies for Arthritis

**Eucalyptus oil:**

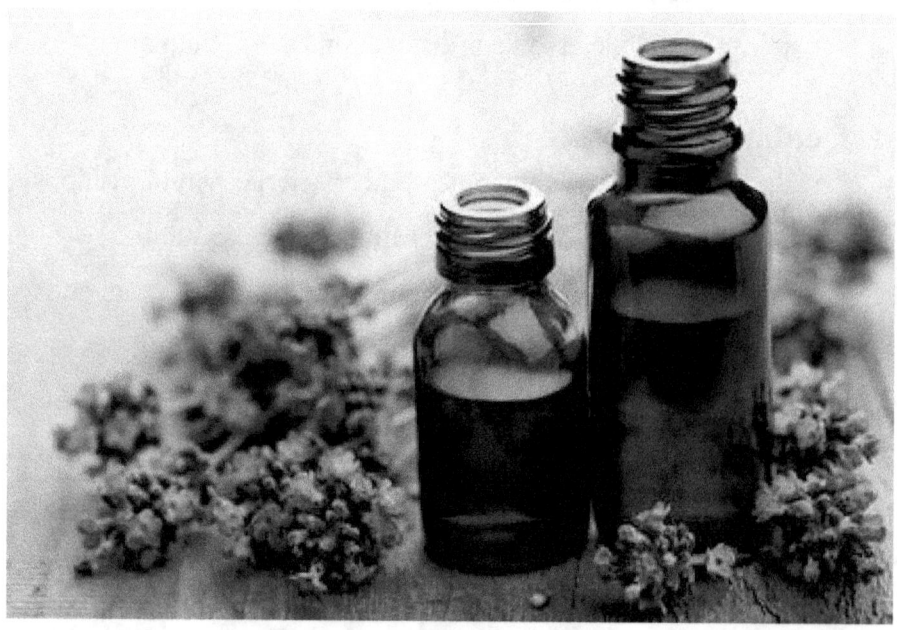

Eucalyptus oil helps in fighting arthritis pain by reducing inflammation. Take eucalyptus oil in small amount and warm it slightly before use. Now, gently massage the painful joint or the painful area with help of this oil. After massaging oil for few minutes, leave it and apply hot compress. Use steaming towels or plastic wrap for this purpose. This method helps in alleviating pain.

## Turmeric:

Turmeric has wonderful power to reduce inflammation associated with arthritis. If you are having joint aches and pain then start treating it with things available in your kitchen. The first thing that comes in mind is turmeric as it has proven to reduce inflammation and pain. Take a glass of milk and mix one tablespoon of turmeric powder in it. Drinking this mixture, daily, helps in fighting pain.

## Epsom salt:

Epsom salt is very effective for the patients of arthritis. This salt has the property of maintaining a normal pH of body and reducing the inflammation. Take Epsom salt and lemon juice and mix them in a cup of water. Having a teaspoon of this mixture daily might help in reducing pain. You can also add some Epsom salt in water before taking bath as it will soothe your body.

## Ginger oil:

Ginger is a natural antioxidant. It has a magical property to reduce the substances which mediate and promote inflammation. Ginger has anti-inflammatory role and is very beneficial for treating the pain and swelling of joints in arthritis. Applying ginger oil on the affected area helps in reducing pain and tenderness.

## Borage seed oil:

Borage seed oil is an effective remedy for arthritis pain. This oil has anti-inflammatory action and helps in reducing pain, swelling and stiffness. Take small amount of borage seed oil and massage it on affected joint. This will help in alleviating pain. You can also take it orally, one tea spoon daily, to get relief from arthritis.

## Cod liver oil:

Cod liver oil is good for people suffering from arthritis. Cod liver oil contains omega 3 fatty acids which are natural antioxidants. Omega 3 fatty acids prevent the formation of reactive oxygen species which are responsible for inflammation. So, when the inflammation is reduced by omega 3 fatty acids, the associated signs of inflammation such as pain, redness, swelling and warmth also get reduced. Take a teaspoon of cod liver oil and mix it in glass of orange juice. Drinking this mixture daily helps you in fighting joint pain.

## Vinegar:

Apple cider vinegar contains vitamin C which is a natural antioxidant. Vitamin C fights against the mediators of inflammation and protects the joints from harmful and damaging effects of inflammation. Applying apple cider vinegar with hot compress helps in relieving pain. Also, take 2 teaspoon of apple cider vinegar, 2 teaspoon of honey and mix them is cup of warm water. Having this mixture once a day is an effective remedy for arthritis.

## Olive oil massage:

Olive oil massage is one of the most ancient remedies for relieving joint pain and aches. Virgin olive oil contains natural antioxidant substances like omega 3 fatty acids which prevent the spread of inflammation and reduce chemical mediators which are responsible for pain. Massaging the painful joint with warm virgin olive oil helps in soothing pain.

## Mustard oil:

Mustard oil is used for massaging the painful joints. Mixture of mustard oil and camphor powder is an effective remedy for arthritis. Massage the affected joint with this mixture twice a day to get rid of pain.

## Cold packs:

Apply cold packs on inflamed joint. Take ice cubes, wrap them in a cloth and place it on painful joint for 15 min. This method is very helpful in suppressing pain and inflammation.

# Herbal remedies for arthritis

## Chamomile tea:

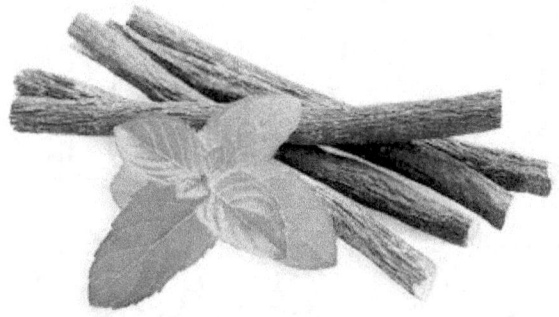

No doubt chamomile is an effective and beneficial herb. That is why it is suggested for the patients of arthritis to drink chamomile tea as it is enriched with natural anti-oxidants which reduce inflammation. To make this herbal tea, mix a tea spoon of chamomile powder in a cup of boiling water. Drink chamomile tea daily if you want to cure arthritis.

## Basil leaves:

Take basil leaves and boil them in water. After cooling the mixture at room temperature, drink it. Basil leaves are helpful in soothing and relieving joint pain by scavenging the free radicals which promote inflammation. Do try this remedy if you are suffering from severe joint pain and are looking for some natural cures.

## Nettles:

Nettle is a very good herb rich in proteins, vitamin A, E, B complex, calcium, phosphorus, iron, magnesium, and silicon. The mineral components of this effective herb are helpful in enhancing the density and strength of bones. In addition, the vitamins present in this herb are very strong antioxidants so they play their role by combating the chemical mediators of inflammation and pain. Tea made from nettles leaves is useful for relieving joint and back pain. Having this tea once or twice a day, helps in relieving the symptoms of arthritis.

## Devil's claw:

One of the most popular and effective herb for relieving back pain is devil's claw. Devil's claw is also known as the natural cortisol (hormone in human body which prevents inflammation by limiting the formation of mediators of inflammation) due to its cortisol like action, it reduces pain by inhibiting the production of prostaglandins and leukotrienes - mediators of inflammation and pain.

## Flaxseed oil:

Arthritis patients must add flaxseed oil to their diet. Flaxseed is enriched with omega 3 fatty acids. Omega 3 fatty acids have anti-oxidant properties and they aid our immune system in fighting inflammation. They relieve pain by limiting the production of reactive oxygen species at the site of inflammation.

## Licorice:

Licorice contains an important component called glycyrrhizin which has anti-inflammatory actions. Licorice acts by blocking inflammation and inhibiting the enzymes which are responsible for the production free radicals. Another important action of licorice is to increase the cortisol production in body. Cortisol inhibits the enzymes and pathway for the production of prostaglandins- mediators of pain and inflammation. Thus pain is relieved.

## Cayenne:

Mixture of cayenne with coconut oil, cocoa butter and lanolin when applied as an ointment on the area of pain is helpful in reducing pain.

## Alfalfa:

Another useful herb for arthritis patients is alfalfa. Alfalfa has the ability to improve circulation and to reduce inflammation. Tea made from alfalfa seeds is healthy and beneficial for arthritis patients. To make tea, take few seeds of alfalfa and boil them in water for few minutes. Drink this tea twice a day if you are seeking cure for joint pain.

## Cinnamon:

Cinnamon has got a magical ability to relieve the joint pain. Take a teaspoon of cinnamon powder and honey and mix it in a cup of warm water. Drink this solution every day to get rid of joint pain. Continuous use of this remedy reduces the attacks of pain in arthritis patient.

## Sesame seeds:

Sesame seeds are suggested to the people suffering from arthritis. They relieve the pain, soothe the joints and make them move with ease. Soak sesame seeds in water for overnight and eat them in the next morning

## Guggulu:

Guggulu is an herb with medicinal importance. This herb is easily available and taking 5mg of guggulu with water, daily, helps in reducing the frequency of arthritis pain.

## Burdock root:

Burdock root has gained importance in the cure of arthritis. This herb is rich in essential fatty acids and oils which are natural anti-oxidants and inhibit inflammation. Dried burdock roots can be chopped to powder and 2 tablespoons are taken daily to relieve pain. Burdock root can also be taken in the form of tea by boiling the roots is water for few minutes and drinking the mixture.

## Dandelion leaves:

Dandelion leaves extract is very effective for reducing the intensity of pain in arthritis. Dandelion juice or tea in morning, regularly, for few weeks helps in curing the arthritis naturally.

# Lifestyle Changes During Arthritis

Your life style and daily routine activities matter a lot in any kind of disease or illness. No doubt when you are not in a good and balanced state of health, it certainly affects your ability to perform day to day tasks. You can make few amendments by bringing changes in your lifestyle which might help you in fighting your illness.

## Lose weight:

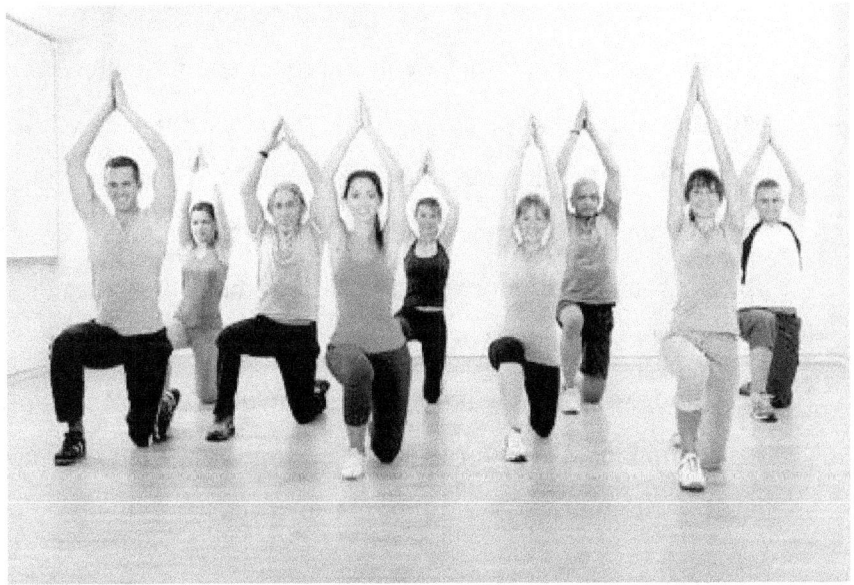

Your joints have capacity to bear stress only to a certain extent. Weight of a person in arthritis is quite important factor.

If you are overweight then you must know that your extra pounds are putting too much strain on your joint, beyond the range of joints to bear it. It has been seen through researches that losing few pounds of weight in patients of arthritis helps in improving the condition. So, all those people who have arthritis and are overweight, they should lose extra fat by doing exercise, jogging, swimming or brisk walking.

## Proper diet plan:

Our diet plan has some connection, either directly or directly, with the severity of our disease. Diet always plays an important role in improving the health of arthritis patients. A healthy and balanced diet helps you in getting control over your disease, to a certain extent. Improper and poor diet or diet with high calories can aggravate the pain crisis in people suffering from arthritis. Some people are food lovers and it becomes a tough task for them to avoid and resist their favorite foods. But you will have to do some compromise on your food habits if you want to get rid of this painful condition. So, things will turn in your favor if you spend some time in making a proper diet plan. Taking suggestion from a nutritionist might be helpful in this perspective

## Stress management:

If you are too much worried and tensed about your arthritis then it is going to make your current situation more painful and worse. People have a misconception that being attacked by a disease make them useless and unfit for any kind of activity. This negative approach towards illness should be corrected. It is a proven fact that taking too much stress aggravates the pain. Many arthritis patients become pessimistic about their illness. It is natural because arthritis compromises your daily routine activities and it reduces your working ability. All these factors cast a negative impression on arthritis patients. It is suggested for such patients to reduce their stress level by managing it properly. You can take following steps to get over with your stress:

- o Take proper rest. 8-10 hours of sleep is good.

- o Try to keep calm and spend more time with your family, friends and neighbours.

- o Do yoga as it's effective in reducing stress.

- o Cognitive behavioral therapies are also helpful.

## Take medicine:

Though stress management and proper diet plan are helpful in curing arthritis naturally. But, it only provide the symptomatic relief. For permanent cure of your disease it's inevitable to eradicate the underlying cause of the problem. So, a proper medical treatment is required to get permanent and long term relief from arthritis. Again here, people have a misconception that home remedies and healthy food habits are enough to treat their condition but they must know the significance of medical treatment.

## Avoid smoking:

Smoking has many health hazards. Apart from damaging your lungs smoking has a negative effect on your whole body. Toxic ingredients of smoke decrease the production of connective tissue in body. So smoking, actually, weakens your bone by inhibiting the deposition if connective tissue in them. So quit smoking if you are suffering from arthritis and joint disorders.

# Physiotherapy Treatment for Arthritis

Physiotherapy holds a great significance and value in the treatment of arthritis. The main aim of this treatment is to improve the mobility of joints by using some physical methods. Physiotherapy is an effective method for curing arthritis as it strengthens joints and tends to reduce the pain.

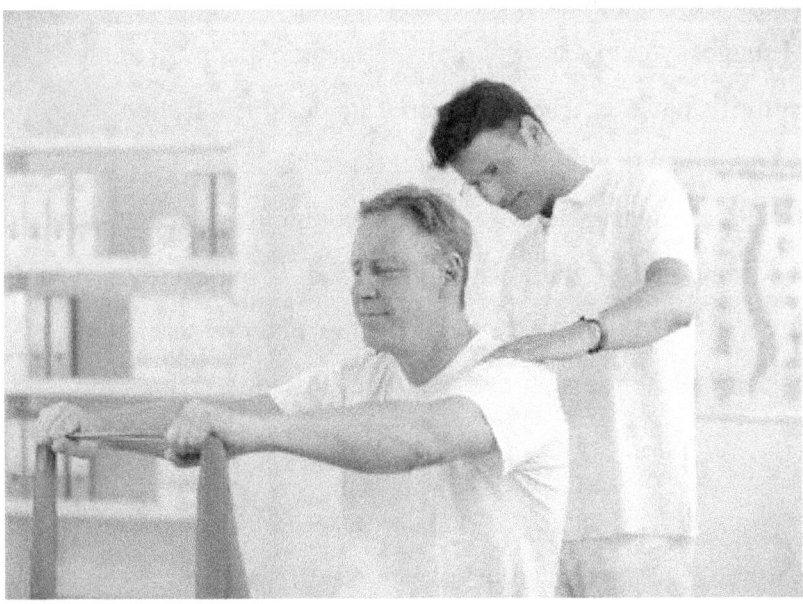

## Massage:

Massaging the joint is the safest and easiest method to get relief from pain. Physiotherapist gives you a light and gentle massage on your painful joints. Massage helps in improving the blood circulation to inflamed joint. As the result, pain is reduced and mobility of joints is increased.

## Physiotherapy exercises:

It is commonly thought that arthritis makes the joints useless and immobile forever and there is no hope of regaining their mobility and flexibility. This wrong concept needs to be changed and modified. Exercise is very important in keeping your joint healthy and mobile. Doing exercise increases the endorphin levels in body which act as analgesics and suppress pain. You must consult a physiotherapist as he'll suggest you exercises which are specific and most appropriate for arthritis patients. These exercises are designed in such a way that they strengthen the muscles and joints and facilitate their ability to move. Precautions must be taken while doing exercises. It is better to first consult a physiotherapist and then start doing exercise. Avoid heavy exercise as they put too much strain and pressure on joints which can further de-stabilize the joints, leading to more pain.

## Exercises to do during arthritis:

For arthritis patients low impact exercises are preferred because they help in making joints more flexible. Some light exercises for arthritis are:

- Low impact aerobics.

- Yoga

- Cycling

- Walking

Exercises to avoid during arthritis:

Heavy and straining exercise can tear the joint ligaments, so they should be avoided.

o Running

o Jumping

o Sports activities

## Hydrotherapy:

Hydrotherapy is technique of physiotherapy which includes water based exercises. In hydrotherapy the buoyancy factor of water is used for exercising. Once you are in water, the body becomes light weighted and the movements of joints are facilitated. Hydrotherapy method has gained importance in the past few years. Physiotherapists are now focusing on it as it is very effective in curing the arthritis pain. The aims of hydrotherapy are:

- To improve blood circulation to joints through exercises.

- To increase the mobility of joint.

- Strengthening of muscles.

- Enhanced flexibility of joints

- Stabilization of joints.

## Electrotherapy:

Electrotherapy is another effective technique for reducing pain intensity in arthritis. The principle of this method is that when electrical stimulus is applied to painful area, it blocks the pain conducting pathways and pain is suppressed. Electrotherapy also raises the level of natural analgesic, endorphins, in body which play an important role in blocking pain transmitting pathway.

# Foods to Eat to Reduce Arthritis

## Fish:

Fish is a very healthy food for people suffering from arthritis. Salmon fish is highly recommended food for joint pain because it contains omega 3 fatty acids which are highly beneficial for health. They have antioxidant properties and support our immune system in getting rid of oxygen free radicals. That is how omega fatty acid reduces pain, swelling and inflammation of joints.

## Soybeans, walnuts:

Walnuts and soybeans are enriched with natural antioxidants like omega 3 fatty acids. They have less caloric content. All those people who are suffering from arthritis must add these contents in their diet.

## Onions

The basic culprit of arthritis and joint pain is inflammation and many chemical mediators produced in body like prostaglandins, leukotirenes, and reactive oxygen radical. All these mediators promote the spread of inflammation and are responsible for severe pain, stiffness and swelling of joints during arthritis. To stop this process foods rich in anti-oxidants should be taken. You do not have to go anywhere to search these foods as they are easily available in your kitchen.

One such food with high content of antioxidants is onion. Onion is helpful in alleviating joint pain and inflammation. So add some extra onion in your daily meal if you want to live a pain free life.

## Green tea

Green tea has several benefits and is helpful in treating various inflammatory disorders. Green tea contains ingredients which are anti-oxidants. They help in reducing inflammation by fighting against the promoters of inflammation. Have a cup of green daily to have a healthy life. Green tea alleviates pain and soothes your body, making it easy for your joints to move.

## Garlic:

Another item found in your kitchen with rich content of antioxidant is garlic. May be you do not like the odor of garlic but still it is effective for minimizing inflammation. Garlic prevents the formation of damaging reactive oxygen radicals by scavenging them. Thus, garlic limits the inflammation and its manifestations like swelling, pain and tenderness. You can add garlic to your daily meal as this will not only enhance the flavor but also helps fight against arthritis.

## Vitamin c rich foods:

Synovial membrane surrounding the joint capsule secretes synovial fluid which provides proper lubrication and facilitates the join movements. The synovium is highly sensitive and its inflammation may lead to decrease production of synovial fluid. As a result, the lubricating mechanism is lost and tearing of cartilages covering the bone starts due to increase in friction. To protect the synovium from damage and inflammation it is suggested to consume foods rich in vitamin C. Vitamin C is a strong antioxidant. Its major role is to prevent the formation of oxygen radicals. Vitamin C deficiency in patients with arthritis can aggravate the situation and make the joint more painful and inflamed. Apart from anti-inflammatory role, vitamin C has a critical role in production and deposition of connective tissue. Vitamin C promotes the production of collagen in bones. Thus vitamin C is necessary for improving the density and strength of bones. Vitamin rich food like,  oranges, grapefruits, mango, cauliflower, lemons and strawberries should be consumed more because they are helpful in reducing pain.

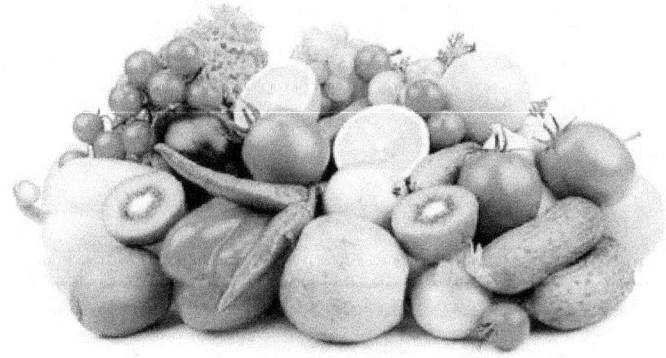

## Selenium rich foods:

Selenium is a mineral present in trace amounts within our body. Selenium has antioxidant role. It is a trace element still it holds a great significance. Selenium levels must be maintained within body to attain protection from oxidizing agents. If you are suffering from arthritis and are on low selenium diet then it's going to worse your joint pain sooner or later. Try to eat selenium rich foods for having healthy bone and joints. Some best foods rich in selenium are Brazil nuts, pasta, oyster, shrimp, whole grains and crabs.

## Carotenoid rich fruits and vegetables:

Many vegetable and fruits are enriched with compounds called carotenes or carotenoids. These are natural anti-oxidants and have the potential to reduce inflammation. The best amongst all carotenes are beta carotenoids. One of the beta carotenes known as beta- cryptoxanthin plays an important role in arthritis. This carotene is specific for arthritis and helps in limiting inflammation induced damage of synovium in patients with arthritis. Foods rich in carotenes are carrots, spinach, broccoli, Brussels, pumpkin, turnips and apricots.

## Foods rich in bioflavonoid:

Flavonoids are natural antioxidant substances present in rich quantity within fruits and vegetable. Flavonoids are vital for preventing the tissues of body from inflammation. These compounds have a protective role in arthritis. Flavonoids prevent the formation of tumor necrosis factor, prostaglandins, leukotienes and cytokines. All of these are inflammatory chemicals and their levels are high in arthritis. Flavonoids, by inhibiting the production of these chemical, reduce the chances of inflammation of synovial membrane. Foods rich in flavonoids are helpful in relieving arthritis pain. Some foods with high content of flavonoids are cherries, raspberries, strawberries, plums and grapes.

## Fish oil and olive oil:

Cooking oils used in routine contain saturated fats which are not good for health especially for arthritis patients. So it's suggested that people having arthritis should stop using these cooking oil and replace them with either fish oil or olive oil. These oils contain high contents of unsaturated fats and essential fatty acid like omega 3 fatty acids which play their role by reducing inflammation and painful condition of joints.

## Avocado:

Avocado contains mono-unsaturated fatty acid which act as antioxidants and serve to reduce pain and swelling. They prevent the irritation and inflammation of synovial membrane.

## Spices:

If you want to cure your arthritis then do add some spice, peppers and chilies in your food. Spices stimulate the production of endorphins in body which act as natural analgesics by blocking pain transmitting neuronal pathways.

So, adding spices and peppers in your food not only enhances flavor of food but also suppresses the joint pain.

# Foods to Avoid During Arthritis

## Red meat:

Red meat is the richest source of proteins. It contains nitrogen containing bases called purines. Breakdown or metabolism of these nitrogenous compounds produces uric acid. Excessive consumption of red meat can elevate the levels of uric acid above normal. High levels of uric acid are toxic and may induce inflammation is joints as seen in gout. So, meat restricted diet might be beneficial for arthritis patients.

## High caloric food:

High caloric and fatty food can aggravate the situation in case of arthritis pain. Consumption of calories more than a limit can lead to increase in weight. This puts burden on joints of body, causing the damage to cartilages and ligaments. So, reduce the intake of carbohydrate rich foods to prevent further worsening of arthritis.

## Nightshade vegetables:

Avoid nightshade vegetable such as tomatoes, potatoes, egg plants and paprika. These vegetables contain high content of alkaloids which may promote inflammation in arthritis patients. So, restrict the intake of these vegetables to get relief from joint pain.

## Gluten:

Gluten is a protein present in wheat. Arthritis patients who are allergic to gluten must avoid its use because gluten can cause inflammation of joints by over stimulating the immune system of body.

## Alcohol:

Alcohol disturbs the generalized health state of a person. Its corrosive action damages the connective tissue and collagen matrix of bones, resulting in weakness and softening. People suffering from arthritis should stop consuming alcohol in order to prevent further loss.

# Allopathic treatment for arthritis

## Analgesics:

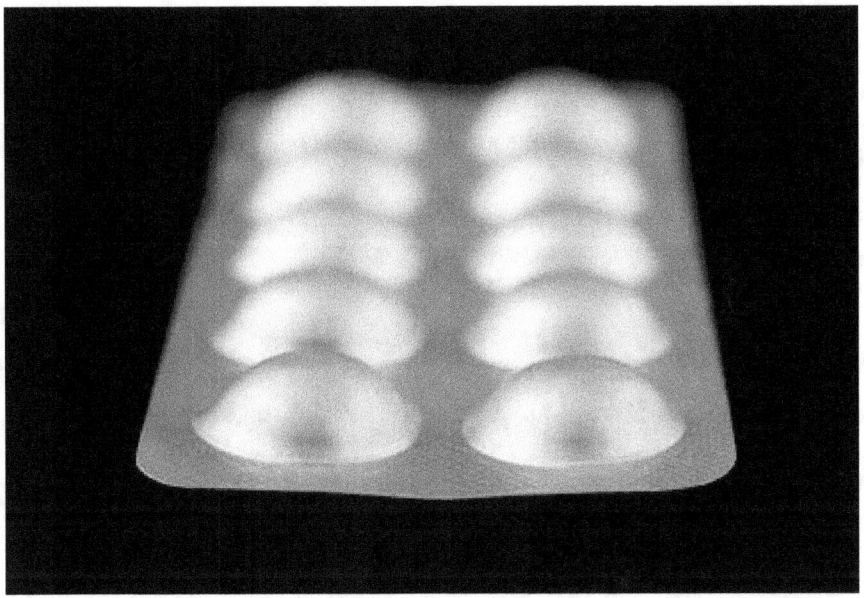

Analgesics are also known as pain relievers. They act by inhibiting the neurons involved in transmission of pain from peripheral areas of body to brain. Analgesics are effective only for pain. They have no role in limiting the inflammation associated with arthritis. Commonly used analgesics are:

- o Acctaminophcn (Tylcnol)
- o Tramadol (Ryzolt andUltram)

Non-steroidal anti-inflammatory drugs (NSAIDs):

NSAIDs are the inhibitors of cyclooxygenase enzyme, involved in synthesis of prostaglandins and other chemical mediators of inflammation. NSAIDs are effective in reducing pain as well as inflammation. NSAIDs are contraindicated in patients suffering from peptic ulcer because they have the ability to exacerbate the ulcer. NSAIDs used for arthritis are :

- Ibuprofen
- naproxen

Corticosteroids:

Steroids are anti-inflammatory drugs. They inhibit synthesis of inflammatory mediators. They can be given orally or injected into affected joint. Prednisone is the most commonly used corticosteroid for arthritis. Steroids are given for long term treatment of arthritis.

Disease modifying anti rheumatic drugs (DMARDs):

DMARDs are the immunosuppressant drugs. They are useful in treatment of auto immune diseases like rheumatoid arthritis. These drugs limit the formation of auto immune antibodies which are responsible for inflammation in rheumatoid arthritis. Examples include methotrexate, minocycline, and hydroxychloroqiune.

# Surgical Treatment for Arthritis

## Total Joint replacement:

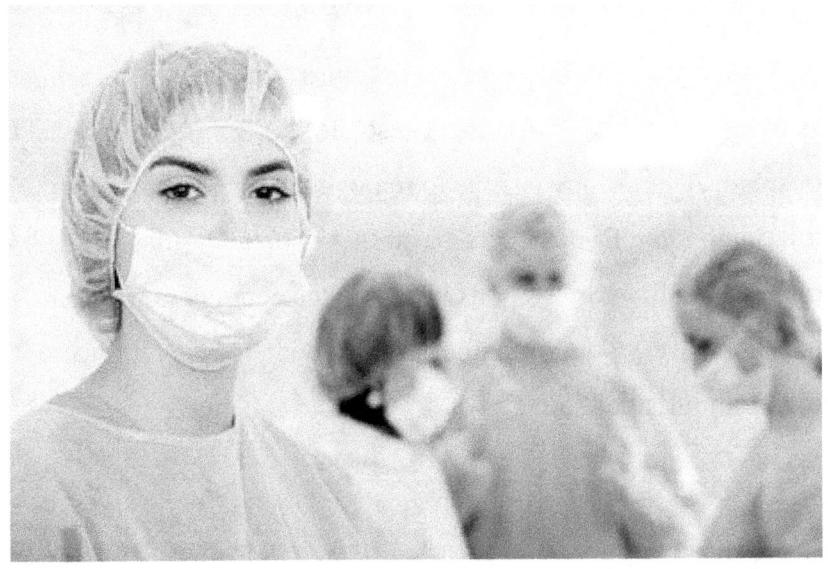

Joint replacement is done when all other medical treatments become ineffective and the only way to cure arthritis is to replace the joint. In this method, surgery is done to remove the worn out parts of bones and joints and are replaced by metallic or ceramic plates. The procedure is usually done in patients who are severely disabled due to arthritis.

## Arthrodesis:

Arthrodesis is the surgical procedure in which torn out and damaged parts of bones and cartilages are removed and the remaining bones are fused together. Bone fusion is followed by regaining the strength of joints. However, the flexibility and mobility of joints is compromised permanently.

## Arthroscopy:

In arthroscopy, a tube like instrument arthroscope is used for surgery. This procedure is less invasive because the surgical incision given is very small. Arthroscopy is done to remove the broken pieces of cartilages in joint. Damaged and worn out parts of cartilages and bone stimulate inflammatory response, leading to accumulation of debris which can be very painful. Arthroscopy is done for the removal of this debris from inflamed joint.

## Arthroplasty:

Arthroplasty means reconstructing of joint. The damaged, rough and worn out part of cartilages and bones are resurfaced in arthroplasty.

## Osteotomy:

In this surgical procedure, the ends of bone are cut first and then re-aligned in a way to give joints more stability and strength. This method is done in young children but it is not very effective.

# Photo Credits

All Images Licensed by Fotolia.com

Full length portrait of a senior man walking with cane

© *LjupcoSmokovski* - Fotolia.com

Young female surgeon with medical team in back before surgery

© *gpointstudio - Fotolia.com*

Fruits and vegetables

© *alinamd - Fotolia.com*


Group of people doing aerobics exercises

© *apops - Fotolia.com*

Licorice and mint

© *scis65 - Fotolia.com*

Gout of the big toe, eps10

© *Alila Medical Images - Fotolia.com*

Backache

© *alphaspirit - Fotolia.com*

## Author Bio

Muhammad Usman is a distinguished medical graduate of Allama iqbal medical college (AIMC). He is a professional writer who has been in the field for more than 4 years. During this time he has produced 10,000+ articles, blogs and eBooks on various niches related to diseases, health, fitness, nutrition and well-being. He is a regular contributor to several journals related to medicine and surgery. He is the editor of several journals and newspapers.

Check out some of the other JD-Biz Publishing books
Gardening Series on Amazon

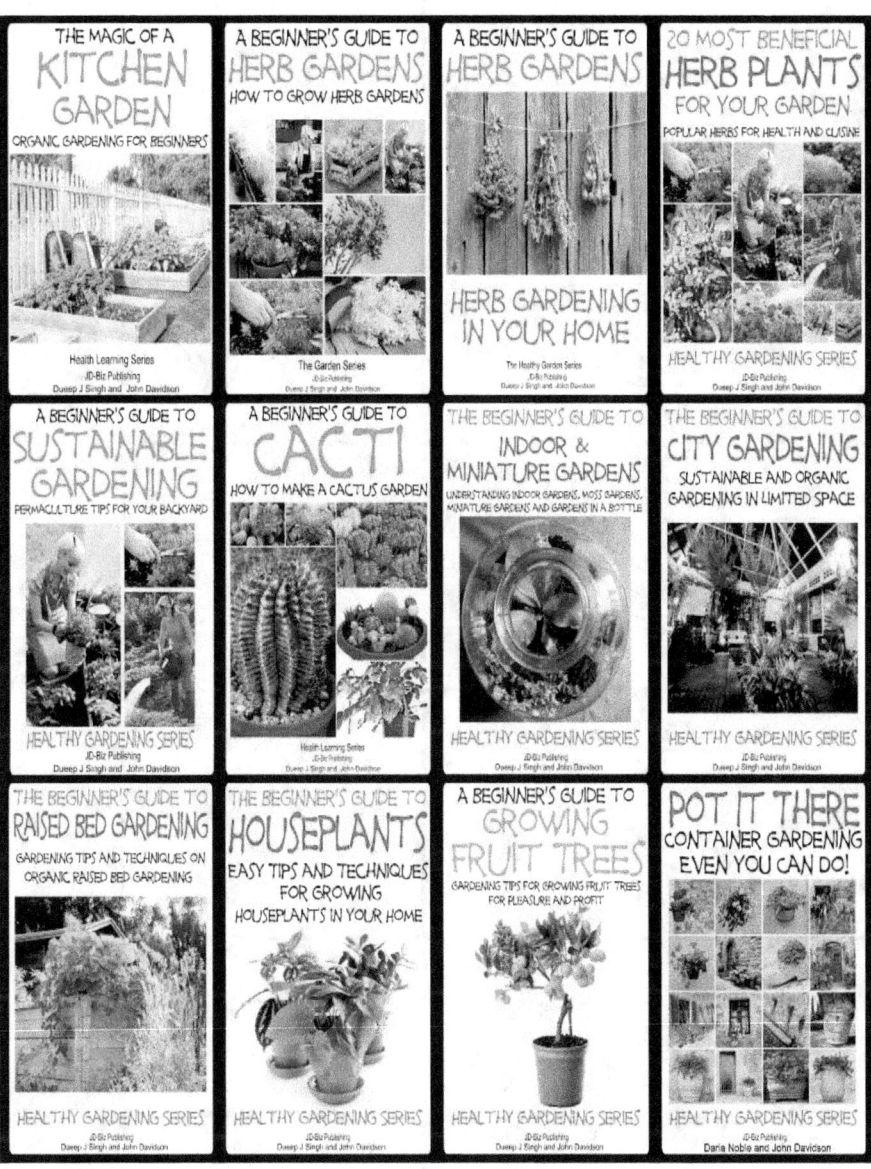

# Health Learning Series

THE MAGIC OF GOOSEBERRIES FOR HEALTH AND BEAUTY

THE MAGIC OF YOGURT FOR COOKING AND BEAUTY

THE MAGIC OF LEMONS USING LEMONS FOR HEALTH AND BEAUTY

THE MAGIC OF CHILLIES FOR COOKING AND HEALING

THE MAGIC OF ONIONS ONIONS IN CUISINE TO CURE AND TO HEAL

THE MAGIC OF RADISHES TO CURE AND TO HEAL

THE MAGIC OF CARROTS TO CURE AND TO HEAL

THE HEALTH BENEFITS OF OREGANO FOR COOKING AND HEALTH

THE MAGIC OF MARIGOLDS Marigolds for Health And Beauty

THE HEALTH BENEFITS OF CINNAMON

THE MAGIC OF COCONUTS FOR COOKING & HEALTH

THE MAGIC OF CLOVES FOR HEALING AND COOKING

THE MAGIC OF ASAFETIDA FOR COOKING AND HEALING

THE MAGIC OF NEEM MARGOSA TO HEAL

THE MAGIC OF SALT TO HEAL AND FOR BEAUTY

THE MAGIC OF POMEGRANATES FOR HEALTH AND BEAUTY

THE MAGIC OF DRY FRUIT AND SPICES REMEDIES AND RECIPES

THE HEALTH BENFITS OF TURMERIC CURCUMIN FOR COOKING AND HEALTH

THE MAGIC OF ALOE VERA

THE MAGIC OF VEGETABLES ANCIENT HEALING REMEDIES AND TIPS

THE HEALTH BENFITS OF ROSEMARY FOR COOKING AND HEALTH

THE MAGIC OF PEPPER & PEPPERCORNS FOR COOKING & HEALING

THE MAGIC OF MILK, BUTTER AND CHEESE FOR COOKING & HEALING

THE MAGIC OF CARDAMOMS FOR COOKING AND HEALTH

THE HEALTH BENFITS OF BLACK CUMIN FOR COOKING AND HEALTH

THE MAGIC OF BASIL-TULSI TO HEAL NATURALLY

THE MAGIC OF SPICES FOR HEALTH AND CUISINE

THE MAGIC OF ROSES FOR COOKING AND BEAUTY

The Miraculous Healing Powers of GINGER

The Miracle of HONEY

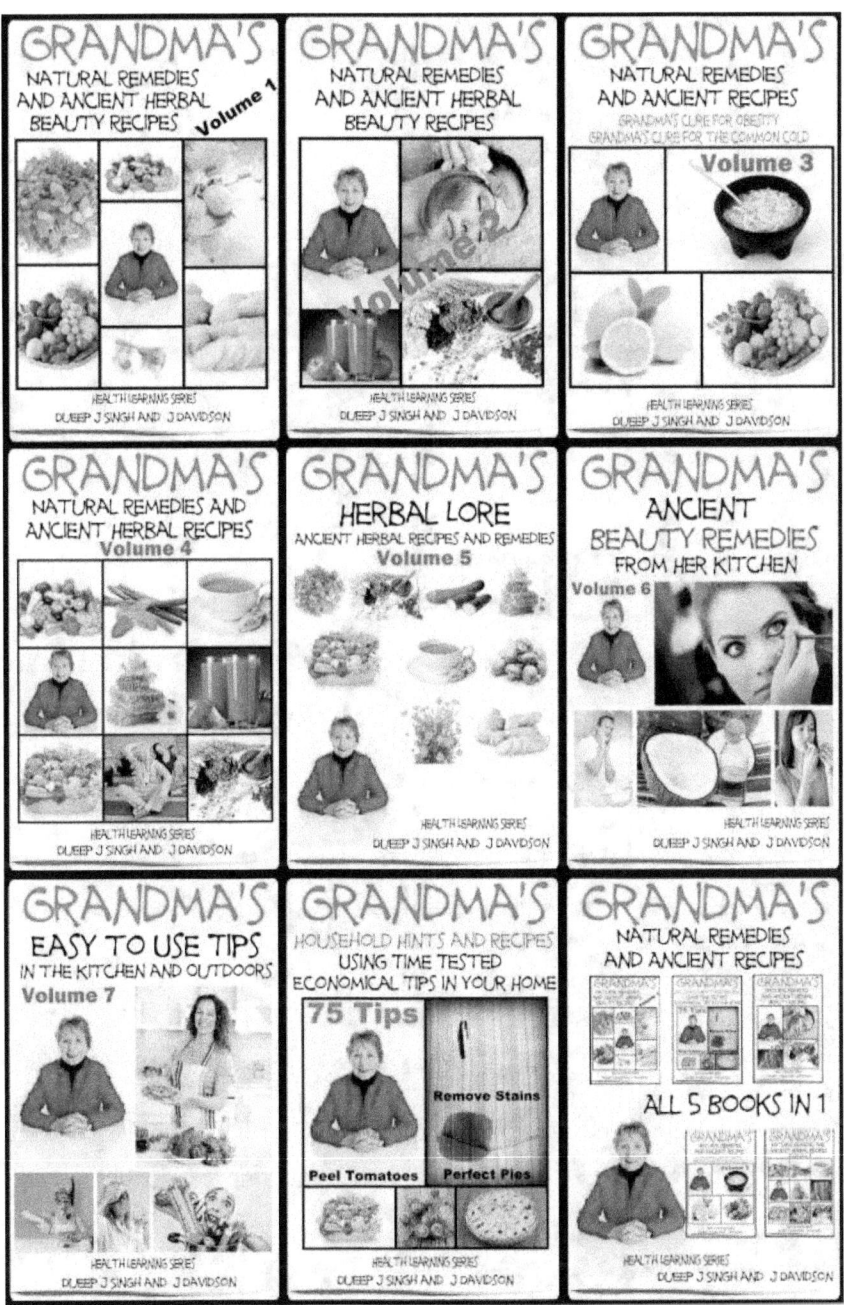

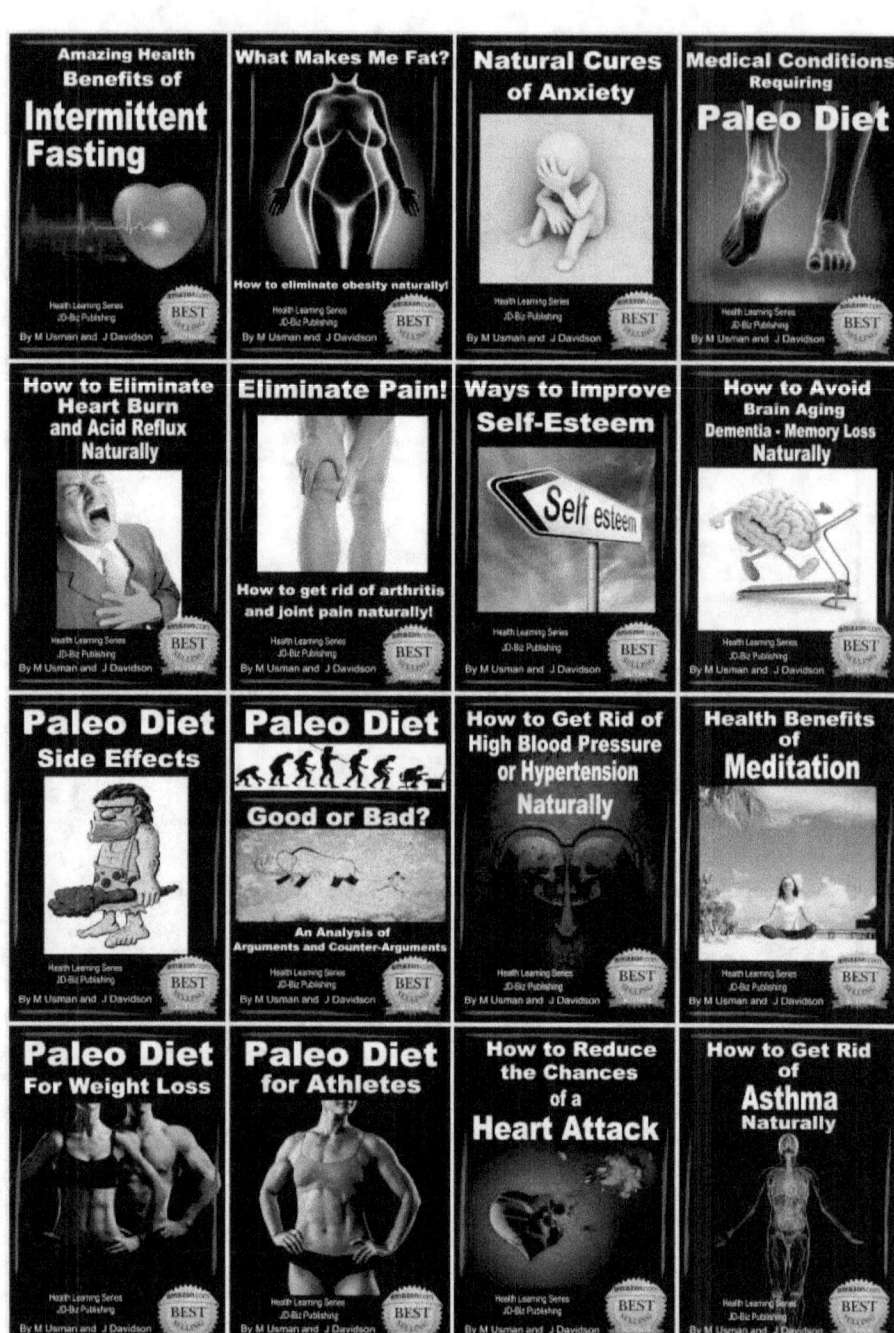

# Amazing Animal Book Series

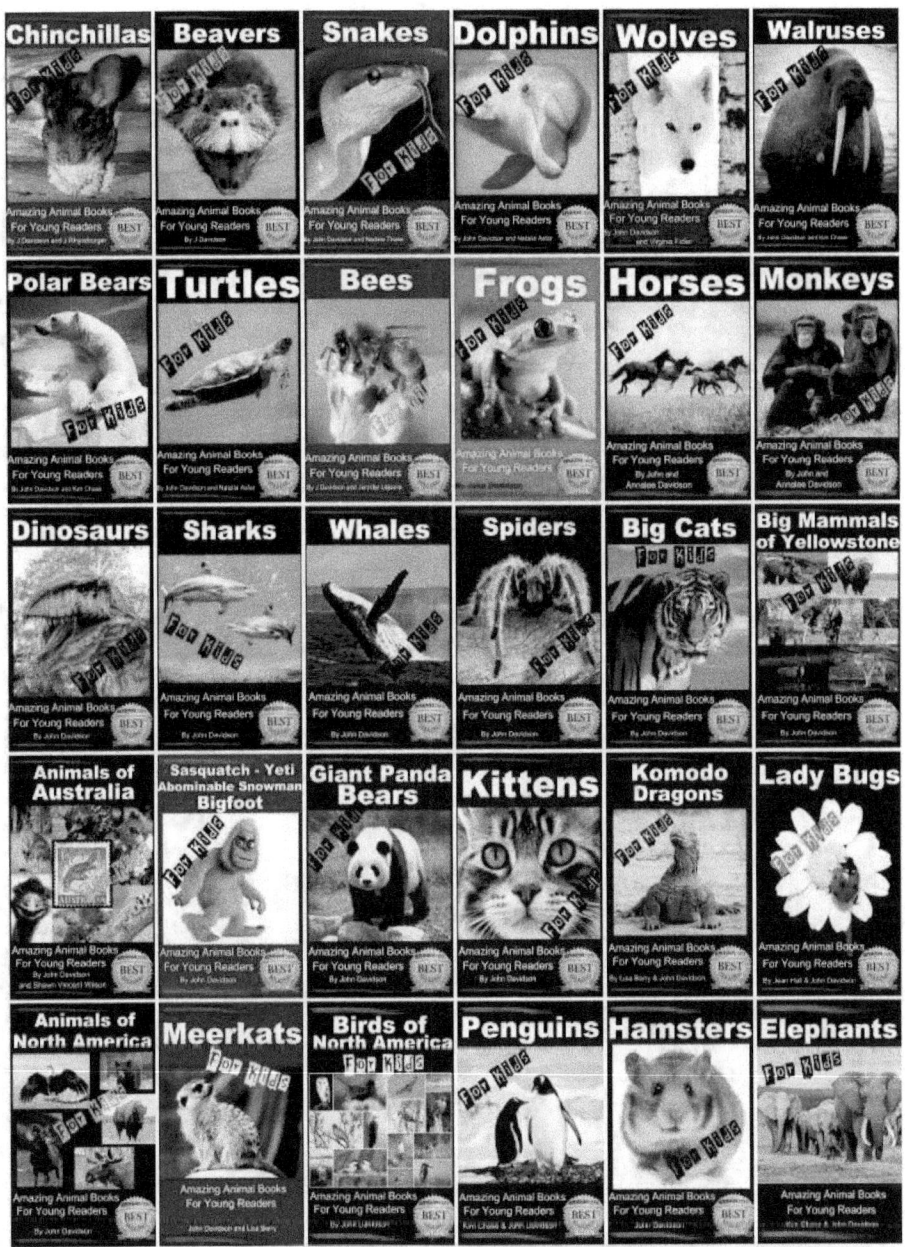

# Learn To Draw Series

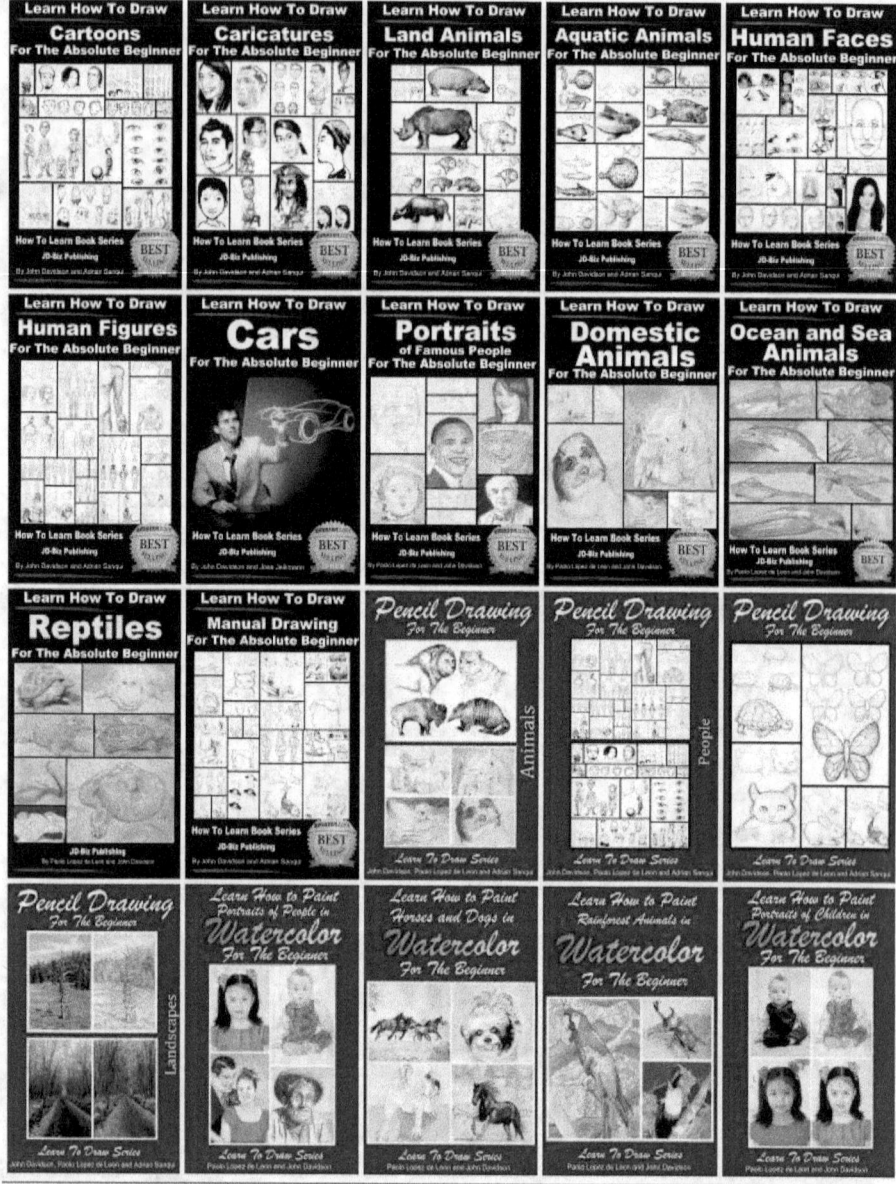

# How to Build and Plan Books

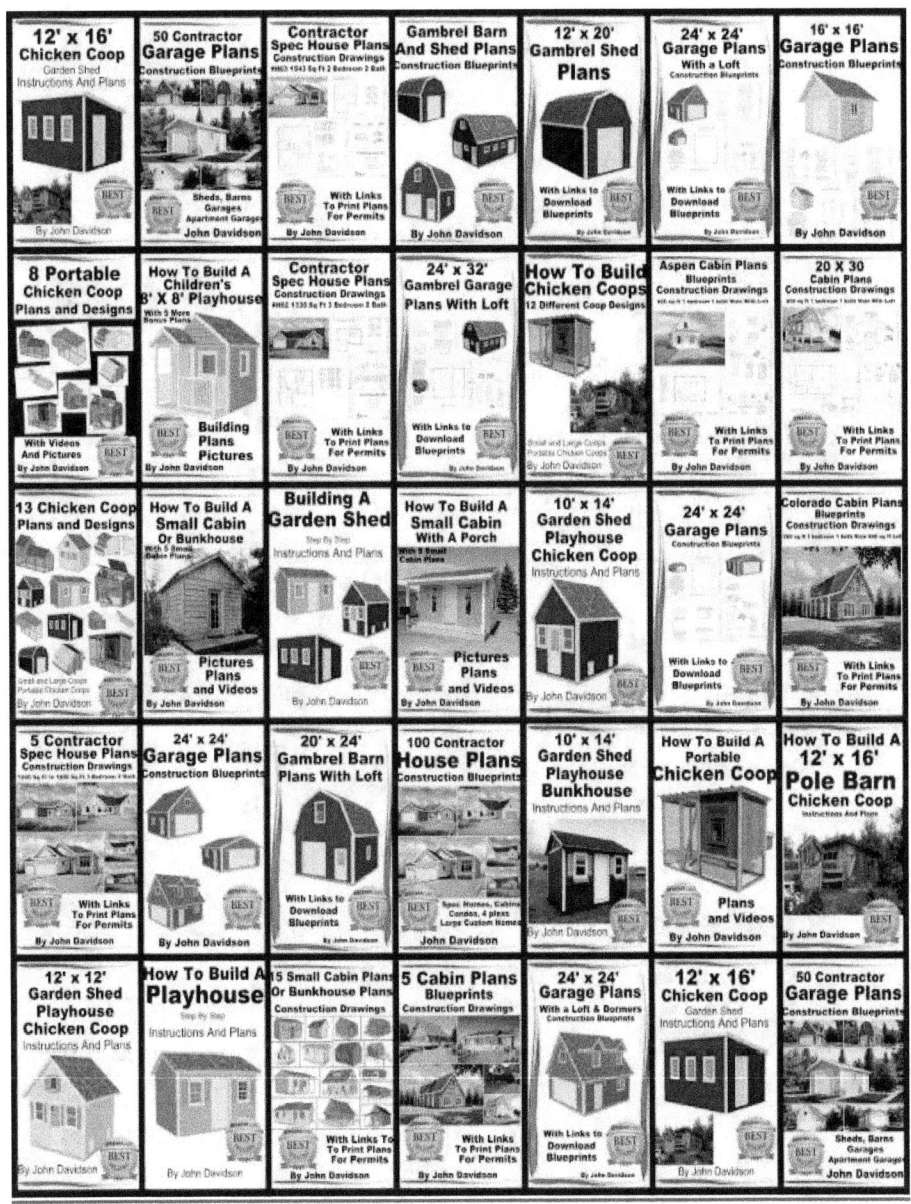

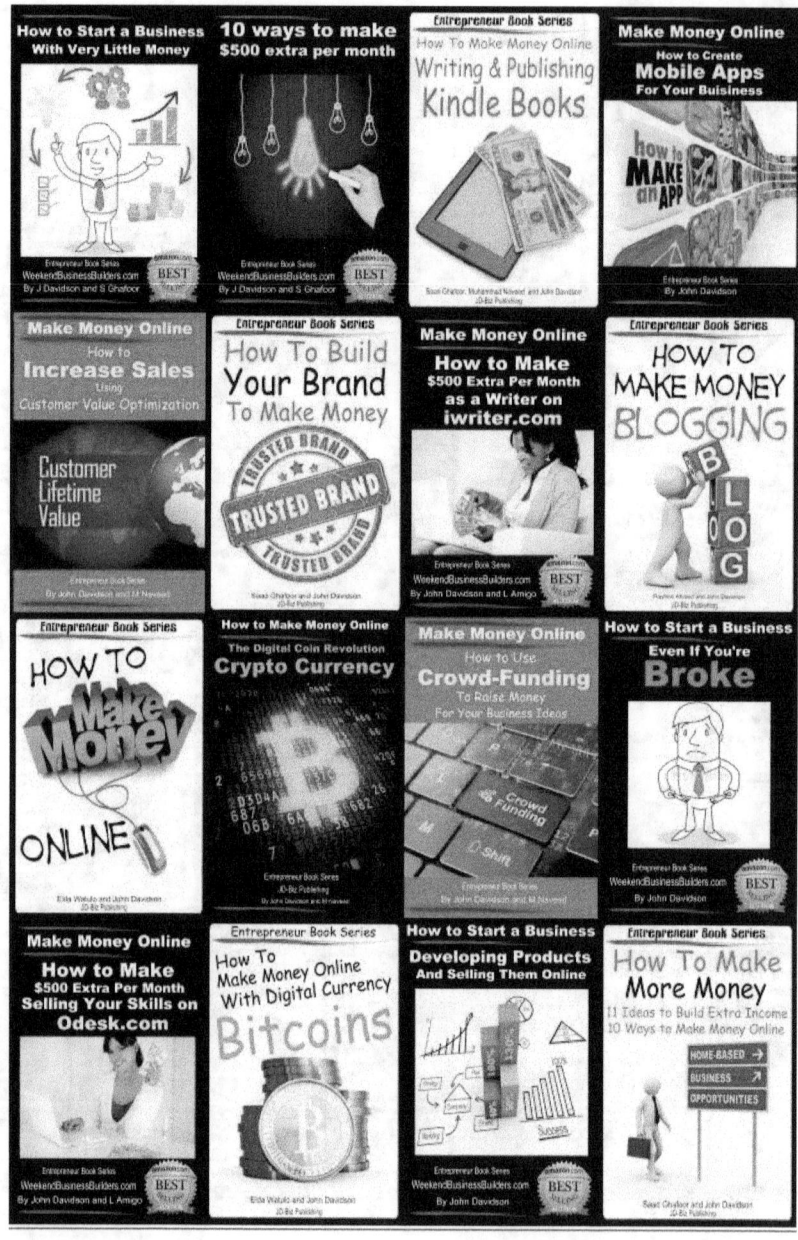

**Our books are available at**

1. Amazon.com
2. Barnes and Noble
3. Itunes
4. Kobo
5. Smashwords
6. Google Play Books

# Download Free Books!
# http://MendonCottageBooks.com

# Publisher

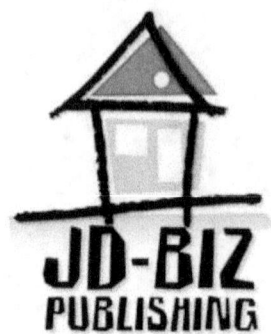

JD-Biz Corp

P O Box 374

Mendon, Utah 84325

http://www.jd-biz.com/

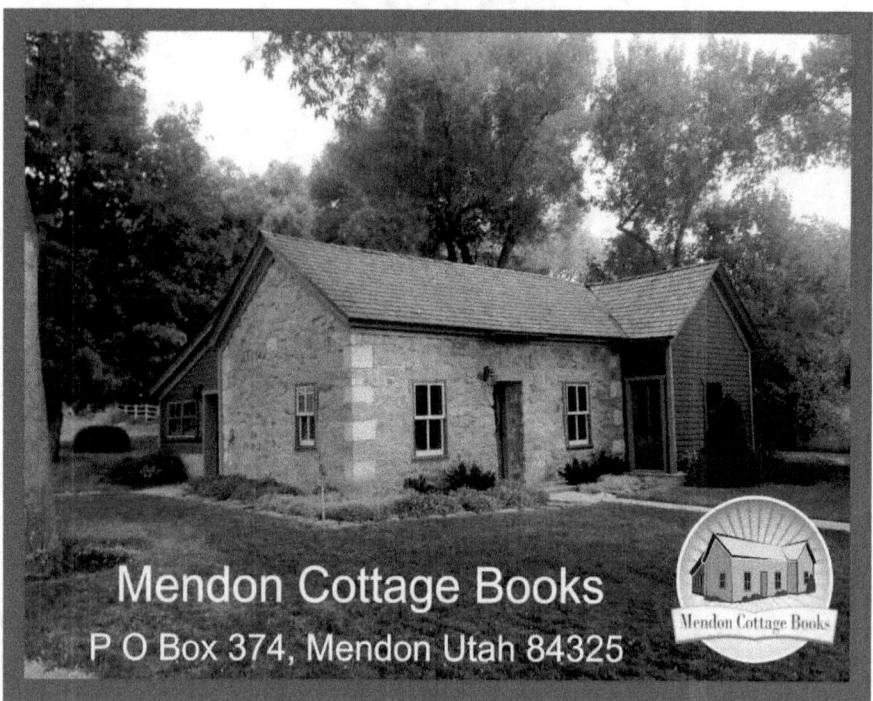